Table of Contents

Preventing Asthma Attacks: A Comprehensive Guide

First Aid for Asthma Attack - With and Without Inhalers

1. Introduction to Asthma

1.1. Definition and Types of Asthma

1.2. Prevalence and Impact

2. Understanding Asthma Attacks

First aid for asthma without an inhaler is given to those who have difficulty breathing or who don't have any other kind of asthma medication; for instance, the inhalers have run out of charge. The patient can take cromolyn or nedocromil in an emergency. No matter how serious the situation, the patient requires immediate medical attention. If the first aid for an asthma attack does not work, or if the patient's condition worsens, such as not being able to walk or talk, seeking medical help should be a priority. Nobody should try to self-medicate or treat asthma sufferers on their own. Anybody who uses high-dose steroids should be taken to the closest healthcare provider right once they start showing symptoms. This can exacerbate symptoms.

Asthma is a condition in which the air passages in the lungs constrict due to inflammation. When a person with asthma is exposed to one or more triggers, they can get asthma attacks, which can get worse in a matter of seconds. The inflammation narrows the channels excessively, causing them to constrict, and mucus production increases, leaving the patient breathless. These factors can add to the severity of an asthma attack. All asthma patients have triggers. As a result, first aid for an asthma attack without an inhaler should be provided to the patient as soon as possible, starting with the symptoms the patient is experiencing. Symptoms might include breathing difficulty, wheezing sound, difficulty to talk, difficulty leaving someone alone, speech difficulty (difficulty speaking in complete sentences), feelings of tightness inside the chest, wheezing that cannot be reduced with medication, breathing rates of more than 25 breaths per minute, exhaling for more than 20 seconds, trouble exhaling.

2.1. Triggers of Asthma Attacks

It is advised that people work to reduce the risk by taking active steps because being able to identify potential triggers can help in avoiding them, thereby reducing the chances of having an asthma attack, according to the American College of Allergy, Asthma, and Immunology. When the airway becomes inflamed, it swells and fills with mucus. The airway muscles also end up being cramped. The resulting symptoms include shortness of breath, wheezing, cough, and chest tightness. Although asthma is a lifelong condition, there are techniques and drugs that can alleviate and manage its symptoms. In some cases, an individual may go for lengthy periods of time without displaying any symptoms. In others, asthma cannot be relieved with medications or can lead to death as a result of therapy. Asthma symptoms can be very severe in these cases. What might also cause an asthma attack in rare cases is a heightened state of excitement.

People with asthma have sensitive airways that can become inflamed when triggered by certain factors, such as cigarette smoke, pollen, or exposure to irritants like household detergents. Asthma attacks can be set off in response to a number of different factors, including, for example, exposure to allergens or viruses. Exercise is another obstacle that sometimes leads to exercise-induced bronchoconstriction and asthma attacks. It's estimated that at least one in every twelve persons who suffer an asthma attack may have an asthma attack because of it. Several asthma attacks and asthma exacerbations require the victim to be transported to the emergency department and, if untreated and severe, may become secondary attacks. It's crucial for folks who have asthma, as well as their caregivers, to recognize what elements can cause an asthma attack and how they can avoid being subjected to these triggers.

2.2. Symptoms and Severity

Managing an acute attack involves addressing both the distress and the bad airflow that underlies the distress. This is bubbles and airways. Crucially, the more bad the airflow – often demonstrated as the air trapping in an FEV1 on spirometry – the worse the air hitting the blood, and the more dead the patient.

Risk The biggest risk from asthma is that the patient can be dead within minutes if the attack turns quickly severe. This is especially true in those who experience pediatric asthma, delving into adulthood. Those who suffer after age 45 are at a minor risk since their airways are less sensitive to bronchospasm. Most deaths occur in people not receiving medical care, poor mental health, or serious attacks in the last 4 weeks.

Severity Asthma attacks can range from very mild to pretty grim. They range from two things – the actual risk of damage and the instant distress. Neither is how bad the airflow is or the wheezing or the 'tightness'. These are signs of airway obstruction, although beware as wheeze isn't everything. An attack is 'severe' if the patient can't talk in phrases. It is assessed on this because a patient's ability to use vocal cords to talk is mediated by cranial nerves, and these show the brain is adequately oxygenated.

Symptoms of asthma attack The mild symptoms of the attack can be like coughing, a tight feeling in the chest, continual wheezing. It can also be sometimes confused with hay fever if mild. The moderate symptoms include symptoms of a mild attack and rapid shallow breathing (tachypnea), faster pulse, sweating, inability to concentrate and talking in words instead of complete sentences, discomforting on bending over (prefers to sit and lean forward on the table). Severe symptoms can present with rapid breathing, use of accessory muscles, hypoxemia, drowsiness, agitation or confusion, chest pain, and cyanosis.

3. Importance of First Aid

The goal of early recognition is to decrease the progression to severe symptoms or, if less severe symptoms are already occurring, to take medications quickly to reduce symptoms and the likelihood of a more severe episode and related healthcare issue. Consider a plan to make sure undertreated people receive support to achieve high-quality clinical care. Emphasizing the need for ongoing clinical care to help people cope with asthma and reducing triggers of an asthma attack and their triggers may be particularly important. That is why continuous professional care and patient education are important in clinical guidelines. Educating people about asthma, including describing an asthma attack and how to recognize and manage its symptoms, is important. Empowering individuals with asthma (or their parent(s)/guardian(s) or other caregivers in the case of children) to manage their asthma and recognize worsening symptoms, as well as providing them with a written action plan, can lead to improved outcomes.

First aid is the provision of initial care for an acute illness or injury. It is usually performed by a layperson to a sick or injured patient until definitive medical treatment can be accessed. The person providing first aid should be aware and equipped to give essential medical care, including early recognition and intervention of the signs and symptoms of an asthma attack. First aid is initiated early by people in the area where an individual has suffered symptoms of the asthmatic condition. Indeed, "The critical intervention in the initial management of an asthma attack is the administration of inhaled β2-agonist bronchodilator; its ultimate role is the prevention of the complications of severe airflow obstruction if possible."

3.1. Early Recognition and Intervention

A few signs of serious asthma can be wheezing, extreme cough, shortness of breath, or a tough time inhaling. Inhaling medications will most likely help you control the symptoms or symptoms if your asthma is under control and you start to encounter new symptoms. Throughout the case that asthma drugs don't help the symptoms or symptoms, an early asthma strike can occur. Strong, hazardous drugs are effective in asthma therapeutic approaches. These are used in cases of serious asthma that endangers a person's life. For the full treatment of asthma, regular follow-up visits are necessary. These consultations can assist you in identifying any underlying asthma path. You may want to explore your alternatives with an allergy professional, who can assist you in understanding the causative variables and starting the necessary maintenance or preventive care.

Early recognition and intervention can prevent discomfort and decrease the severity of an asthma attack. Asthma triggers can be anything from the flu or cold to a pet's fur, but inflammation and swelling in the air passages are always being stopped. Spasms or contractions of the sinews - circular muscles surrounding the lungs - are also blocked. These factors reduce the amount of air a person can breathe into their lungs, causing asthma symptoms. Shortness of breath, a gripping discomfort in the thorax, tiring very readily, coughing, and wheezing are all frequent symptoms. Inhaling drugs can help open the airways if a person feels tight in the chest. These are the primary and most effective means of asthma management.

3.2. Role of First Aid in Preventing Complications

The proactive first aid approach is to make use of medications such as inhalers to stop asthma attacks. For example, administration of a metered-dose inhaler with albuterol during the first signs of an asthmatic attack and cetirizine and loratadine which are first-generation antihistamines especially during the allergic phase or flu phase has been proven effective in preventing asthma attacks. Inhaled corticosteroids have to be taken regularly even in legume allergy conditions.

Asthma first aid possesses a two-pronged approach and one has to be proactive if an individual is known to be suffering from asthma. The first proactive approach shall be to avoid known allergens and irritants. This can be achieved by avoiding unhealthy habits such as smoking. There are a number of medications and inhalers that can be used to control asthma but talk to a doctor first. Second, one has to be ready to administer first aid in case of an asthma attack.

Asthma is an ailment wherein the airways get narrowed, swollen, and produce additional mucus. These features make inhalation a tough task and result in coughing and wheezing. Severe asthma attacks can be life-threatening if not taken care of promptly. For that reason, asthma first aid is very important and needs to be administered within the stipulated time. First aid can be the difference between life and death in severe asthma attacks. Attacks can occur at any place and any time. The role of first aid is to help in preventing complications till professional help arrives.

4. First Aid Techniques with Inhaler

B. Steps for using a Metered Dose Inhaler with Spacer: - Shake the inhaler well. - Assemble the spacer with the inhaler. - Remove the cap from the inhaler. - Hold the inhaler with the mouthpiece at the bottom and your thumb pointing to the top. Tilt the head slightly back and breathe out gently. - Place the inhaler in your mouth between your teeth without biting. Close your lips tightly around the mouthpiece so that a good seal is formed.

A. Steps for using a Metered Dose Inhaler without Spacer: - Shake the inhaler well. - Remove the cap from the inhaler. - Hold the inhaler with the mouthpiece at the bottom and your thumb pointing to the top. Tilt the head slightly back and breathe out gently. - Place the inhaler in your mouth between your teeth without biting. Close your lips tightly around the mouthpiece so that a good seal is formed. - Press down on the inhaler while breathing in deeply and slowly. Press the inhaler only once otherwise, it would lead to taking drug out of the inhaler if it is pumped into the air. - Hold your breath for 5-10 seconds and then breathe out very gently.

First aid with inhaler – Metered Dose Inhaler: The prescribed reliever inhaler is the first aid in asthma attack situations. Always use a spacer with a face mask or mouthpiece for inhalers. A spacer device must be used by all those who are not able to coordinate well while using the inhaler and those who have moderate to severe asthma. A metered dose inhaler delivers a specified amount of medication through the inhaler mouthpiece. Such an inhaler must be used very carefully and can be done in 4-8 doses every 20 minutes during asthma attacks, followed by four puffs every 4-6 hours till medical help in the hospital is reached. A metered-dose inhaler delivers a constant amount of medicine in every puff. Asthmatics must take some reliever inhaler dose before starting the nebulizer as it delivers medicine over a period.

4.1. Types of Inhalers for Asthma

Dry powder inhaler (DPI) releases medication in the form of a powder rather than a mist pressed out by a chemical propellant. DPIs are breath-activated, i.e. the patient only has to begin a fast and deep breath-in to get the released medication into the lungs. A direct inhalation device (DID) releases medication when a blister or capsule is inserted and pierced. The medication is actuated directly by the patient's breath. Pen-type inhaler (PI) is a medical device extending from a syringe-like apparatus adapted for use as a metered-dose inhaler for administering medication. It releases medication using a cartridge containing the medication. The handheld nebulizer is an electronic device to release medication in the liquid mist form for breathing in. Most often, portable nebulizers are either piston pumps or vibrating mesh technology types.

In the management of asthma and the asthma attack, several types of inhalers are available. These vary in the medication and the propellant used, and the administration method. The pressurized metered-dose inhaler (pMDI) is a commonly used inhaler, which contains a canister filled with medication in a liquid suspension solution. Most pMDI inhalers are a combination of an asthma reliever medication (for fast-acting relief) and a corticosteroid inhaler (for asthma control). To get the medication from the inhaler into the lungs for asthma management, an HFA-propellant in the canister is activated as a propellant to create medication mist, and the patient coordinates a deep and slow breath to get the misted medication to enter the lungs. A spacer or valved holding chamber helps in situations when the patient cannot coordinate the device correctly. Breath-actuated pressurized metered-dose inhaler (B-pMDI) is similar to pMDIs, except they are designed to release a puff of medication when the patient starts to breathe in.

4.2. Step-by-Step Guide for Using Inhaler

You may often feel a very fine dust or taste in your mouth.

1. Shake well. 2. Breathe out gently to empty the lungs. 3. Inhale the medication in the middle of a gentle breath. This is the most difficult part of the pMDI technique. 4. After inhaling the medication deeply into the lungs, hold your breath for only 2 seconds - any longer can stir up the bronchial tubes (airways). 5. Breathe out gently. 6. Replace the mouthpiece cover and store the pMDI carefully.

Step-by-step guide on how to use an Accord Non-Metered Dose Inhaler (pMDI):

N.B. Sometimes people may not be able to breathe in quickly enough to empty the turbuhaler. If this happens, they can breathe in deeply and then breathe out forcibly in order to inhale the medication.

You may often feel a very fine dust or taste in your mouth.

1. Shake well. 2. Breathe out gently to empty the lungs. 3. Put the mouthpiece in your mouth and close your lips around it. 4. Breathe in quickly and deeply through the inhaler (not your nose), and then remove the inhaler. 5. Hold your breath for as long as is comfortable. 6. Breathe out gently. 7. Replace the mouthpiece cover and store the inhaler carefully.

Step-by-step guide on how to use an inhaler - dry powder:

5. First Aid Techniques without Inhaler

First Aid for Asthma Attack – What You Can Do To Help A Person During An Asthma Attack Make sure that you keep the area around the person having an asthma attack clear of any triggers like dust, smoke, or pollution. Sit the person down in a comfortable position. Some people with asthma may be advised by their GP to take anti-inflammatory medicines called preventer inhalers. If that person's inhaler is with them and you have access to it, help them to take it as prescribed. If the person doesn't feel any relief, then the person can take one or two puffs of their reliever inhalers every two minutes for up to 10 puffs. Sit with them as they take the inhaler or medication. If the person does not feel relief after 10 puffs or if you are in any doubt, call for an ambulance or seek emergency medical help. Do not leave the person on their own. It is important that the person is assessed by a doctor as soon as possible. If There Is No Inhaler Available, if there is no inhaler with the person having an asthma attack or if you haven't used the inhaler in the past, then follow these first aid steps: First Aid Techniques without Inhaler Ask the person to sit up and try to take long, steady, deep breaths. Stay calm and reassure the person. Keep giving them the reassurance until they begin to feel better.

First Aid for Asthma Attack – If There Is No Inhaler Available First Aid for Asthma Attack – What to Do If Someone Is Having an Asthma Attack

First Aid for Asthma Attack – What to Do If Someone Is Having an Asthma Attack First Aid for Asthma Attack – What You Can Do To Help A Person During An Asthma Attack What You Need To Do

5.1. Positioning and Comforting the Person with Asthma Attack

a. Patient position: Somebody having difficulty breathing should be encouraged to sit up because when lying down there is the chance of restricting breathing; in very severe anaphylaxis, where blood pressure drops, this rule does not apply. A comfortable sitting posture with slight forward lean can make breathing easier. Care should be taken when moving someone with an asthma attack; they are at a higher risk of also having a heart attack. An emergency call number for an ambulance should be dialed wherever someone with an asthma attack is unresponsive and not breathing normally. Each year in Australia, there are thousands of deaths from heart attacks, but it is estimated that less than half of the people with symptoms actually use the emergency call number.

5.1. Positioning and comforting the person with asthma attack If a person is experiencing an asthma attack and you are waiting for the ambulance to arrive, there are a few general measures you can take to help the person. As mentioned above, these are aimed at the safe and open airway. It can be very scary for someone to have an asthma attack, even for the 4.8% of Australians who have it every day. As a first-aider, your role is to keep calm and take any efforts to relieve their fear by confidently and calmly performing first aid. These measures are also important because they have been shown in several laboratory studies to increase the amount of air that people can blow out of their lungs in the first second of forced exhalation.

First aid for asthma attack – with and without inhalers

5.2. Encouraging Slow Breathing Techniques

The anti-inflammatory and bronchodilatory effect of inhaled corticosteroids is one of the reasons for its use as a first-line treatment in asthma. A national inquiry into asthma deaths found that most asthma deaths could have been avoided if patients had received appropriate inhaled corticosteroids or had been taken to an emergency department. Using an inhaler may be required for any person with asthma in this condition. Slow breathing in is thought to maximize the amount of perfluorocarbons that are taken into the alveoli, as the gas is denser than air and takes longer to get lower down in the lungs and then stay there, reducing or limiting the discomfort caused by PFC causing a cold shock to alveoli, causing discomfort in larger airways. Administering the combination drug Peskynd or Berodual drop and stationary belt are the first balm to treat or provide responses or urgent reactions in the nozzle of the first four-step method developed by the chest physician Professor Konstantin Pavolovich Buteyko and colleagues at the research laboratory of rehabilitation and posturology at the eye clinic institute in Moscow. Administering bronchodilator in colloidal gas is the only treatment, first aid or otherwise, for asthma attacks, altered states of breathing, and symptoms related to smooth muscle problems in the branches and bronchioles of the trachea, or in responsive disorders such as asthma. Citation needed. Because it rubs and has the consequences of the condition when the causative pathways of asthma dominate the effectual or sympathetic or adverse cause to be able to the division of a member. Immediate response to treatment or administration is vital, as bronchodilator actions can be achieved within seconds or in a maximum of 5 minutes. Inability or unwillingness to inhale from the gas supply cylinder introduces a therapeutic obstacle to overcoming the airways that are narrower. Inability to inhale from glassware containing inhaled corticosteroids is due to the above working in gel form, which is resistant to being blown into the lung so that it can be placed in a large chamber before being 'huffed and puffed' into the top part of the chamber, which comes from the researchers mentioned in the text.

5.2.1 Effects

During the initial treatment or before or during administration of bronchodilator in colloidal drops, the rescuer may encourage the casualty to regulate his or her breathing by using slow breathing in and slow deep exhalation techniques. This method could be discussed with chest physicians to gain their views and the evidence that this technique could be effective and deemed to be safe. Hyperventilation averts hypercapnia caused by airway closure artificially inflating the lungs with the patient's air. Hyperventilation forms part of the Buteyko method of breathing, which can alleviate asthmatic symptoms and is one of its main health interventions.

5.2 Encouraging slow breathing techniques

6. When to Seek Emergency Medical Help

When to Seek Emergency Medical Help.

4. You feel very dizzy standing or sitting up and will faint imminently, if you have not already done so.

3. The exhaustion is so deep that almost no consciousness or alertness remains – the person is almost in a coma and cannot be woken easily or at all. In other words, it may be difficult to wake up someone whose usual habit is to sleep excessively, but drowsiness from over-sedation does not count.

2. You keep walking into walls and falling over.

1. The breathing is no longer audible. Any efforts to breathe in are either very quiet, or seem to have no effect. You observe a silence period within the effort to breathe, some of the time. This type of no-breath sound is referred to as a silent chest, but no instruments to measure breathing sounds or chest abnormalities are usually available.

- A blue face (cyanosis), suggesting severe oxygen depletion (medical term – hypoxemia) - A drowsy, confused, or agitated, but exhausted, mental state - A collapse - All medications and inhalers are used but there are no signs of improvement. The usual medications and the usual inhaler doses can be taken up to 6 to 10 times. White out

If any of the following symptoms have begun to set in, one needs to seek emergency medical assistance for urgent treatment:

• You have finished in less than 4 hours and the symptoms keep getting worse. Difficulty in breathing, speaking, walking or changing position is increasing. Or, exhaustion has started to set in.

3. Take slow, steady breaths (in and out). Do not: obstruct the person's inhaler, give them your medicines, lie them down giving it as lying down can make it harder for them to breathe effectively, tell them to take deeper breaths, as this will likely make the problem worse, give them strong coffee. You are giving too many close, spaced-out puffs of reliever when the person is not improving or if you're worried at any time, help the person to take to the emergency medical help. Your asthma attack is cleared after the main asthma symptoms go away with the help of relievers. Then further, they could have an off-the-shelf asthma attack in the next few days. To protect this from happening, a GP will usually care for someone who's had an asthma attack.

2. Sit up straight, even if they're struggling to breathe.

1. The reliever isn't working. Ask if they have a reliever inhaler. If they do, ask them to take one puff every 30–60 seconds, up to a maximum of 10 puffs.

If you see any of these signs or if people are still worried even after they use their reliever inhaler, they might be having a life-threatening asthma attack. They will need urgent help. If the situation is becoming worse, make sure someone calls emergency help if they are not already on their way.

6.2. Contacting Emergency Services

If Alone, Make a Quick Decision – If and when breathing becomes significantly more difficult, and the reliever medication does not change the breathlessness in a couple of minutes, quickly take the mobile and call the local hotline number, and provide the required information asked for over the phone and take advice on the best bring-the-patient-to-hospital measure under the circumstances. For a more advanced medical situation, contact the emergency services and request the relevant assistance.

Follow Health Action Plan – A personal emergency health action plan can guide the relative or the caregiver with appropriate and timely medical treatment. If there is difficulty in breathing, ask the caregiver to check whether the casualty is still breathing or not. A clear sign of absence of breath is lifelessness, or the casualty is not responding to speech or touch. Set the casualty in a comfortable position, to reduce physical stress and damage any further. If the casualty is unconscious but still breathing, gently turn the casualty onto his/her side and support the side with his/her upper arm and thigh.

Be Calm – A relative or a friend must support you to understand the situation better. Do not panic at any time. Follow the steps mentioned in the emergency health action plan.

Pack a First Aid Kit – A first aid kit contains essential first aid supplies for any kind of urgent medical situation. This portable trauma pack should ideally be customized according to the severity of one's health. Severe asthma attacks require different components in a first aid bag than moderate episodes. Always include the medication one carries, his/her emergency contact details, inhaler and spacer, preventer medication, reliever inhaler (albuterol), and health action plan.

If you are asthmatic, severe symptoms of asthma can manifest when you least expect it. For this reason, it is always wise to be prepared for worst-case scenarios. Contacting appropriate emergency services can significantly improve your outlook and shorten the duration of your recovery period. Critical steps to take to ensure seamless and timely emergency services include:

7. Preventive Measures and Long-Term Management

Education should improve this score during 2020 and 2022 when commenced October 2020; one year after the PHE requirement and three and a half years into the campaign. Let the unknowns be filled with the necessary information. The most important education is the one you have yet to engage with. However, factors that need the most attention are inhaler management for those attending the review, ensuring that people have an in-date AAP, and exploring their use to prompt attendance for review for those not in-date beyond the usual triggers suggesting a review would be useful. The income from this education justifies the cost of a dedicated review at three levels utilizing outcomes known to be influenced by attending a review. Educational programs specifically aimed at these need the least publicity at present.

Preventive measures and long-term management (Acknowledge) - Avoid the triggers, the most important preventive measure. Almost all recoveries are short-lived or illusory without the avoidance of the triggers. People are encouraged to seek help to identify their triggers with more aggression (Seek and Engage). Ignorance is no one to blame because different people behave differently to an actual threat. The receipt of an asthma action plan (AAP) has been identified by the BTS/SIGN as the least participants of an asthma review. This was all the scores near the bottom. It is likely the first score the doctor or nurse is likely to review.

7.1. Medication Adherence and Asthma Action Plan

Asthma Action Plan (or Bts Asthma Action Plan): The development of an asthma action plan is one of the first things you can do to start taking control of your asthma. It is a written plan that an individual with asthma develops to help control their condition and reduce emergency room or doctor's office visits. The asthma action plan involves identifying triggers and formulating the avoidance of these triggers, the use of medications, the practicing of pulmonary smugglers, and immunization plans. It gives a guide on how to recognize when the asthma is getting out of control (when will it be relevant to consult or report to the hospital). This is a class academic manifestation and the severity of the mode of asthma. A proactive relationship with consideration and recognition of the individual differences and specificity with the trigger factors, exposure, perceptions, beliefs is crucial in asthma control.

Medication Adherence (or Medication Compliance): Medication adherence is defined by the World Health Organization as the degree of conformity by a patient to any medication recommended by their health adviser. Effective use of medications requires that people follow their diagnostic and therapeutic plans thoroughly, thus referring to the clinical practices such as the extent to which a person's medications are taken as prescribed in an effort to improve asthma management. People who take their medications as prescribed to keep their asthma under control will tend to have better controlled asthma. So, a well-crafted explanation on the disease, management with proper classification, the need for long-term management medication, the use of rescue inhalers, side effects of steroid medicine, dose, time, duration, route of administration, and information about the preventers and relievers will be helpful. This understanding can make a person adhere more to the treatment, thus reducing the amount of preventable exacerbations.

7.2. Identifying and Avoiding Triggers

Environmental control produces one of the most cost-effective areas of asthma care. While the history will often give the most important information, proven sensitivity by objective tests, e.g., RAST, proves that the identified factor is a precise trigger. Once it is identified, then if really practical, it may be helpful to suggest to the family that they take steps to avoid it. However, hypersensitivity to aero-allergens is common, and proven hypersensitivity to a particular allergen should be part of overall management and not just an emphasis on environmental control. This may not be practical, e.g., to avoid pet animals in certain patients who have significant pet animal allergies and have had pet animals. Therefore, common sense as well as available data, such as a negative controlled trial of specific avoidance measures in children who are otherwise well controlled on appropriate treatment, should be applied. Environmental control is about exclusion as well as ongoing, long-term prevention and therefore should be a key part of education.

A convenient way to identify asthma triggers is by keeping a diary of daily events, including triggers encountered and an assessment of symptoms. This approach provides a convenient, unobtrusive way of collecting the most important information. In older children, it will help to teach them about the most important triggers and strategies for dealing with them. It is also useful for assessing the child at every health visit and enabling children and parents to become involved in asthma management.

8. Conclusion

The issue of asthma can be understood by a teen for understanding about asthma in trivial barriers of life. The symptoms and the medication for the asthma attack are necessary. Writing a rule notebook by the specialist for keeping it safe in the hands and pockets for making the cure better through the first aid kit. The adults can understand that the respiratory disorder asthma is open to life barriers at any age. It is a challenging condition and it does not limit activities and good health. Eventually, it also suppresses outdoor activities. It finally highlights the limitation of exercise and degrades condition more and more in daily activities. Consult a specialist for curing asthma. It can be tried with medicines and medications. Encourage and convince yourself that it can be cured. Get ready with the following information for managing the first aid for an asthma attack.

People suffering from asthma carry inhalers at all times to be safe and to immediately treat the asthma attack or symptoms of asthma. It is important to control the trigger factors which lead to the asthma attack. People with severe asthma or who suffer from asthma attacks whenever there is no inhaler with them and there is no available hospital should be taken special care of. It becomes very important to treat the primary or first symptoms of an asthma attack naturally or by some remedies. The guide here is for first-aid for the severe attack of asthma with the things you need to feel comfortable. You don't need any other preparations. So, follow the first-aid quickly for the first 5-10 minutes. The effect is felt very fast. People who are not diagnosed with asthma should undergo tests and research. People with asthma attacks, with or without inhalers, are suggested to consult a specialist of asthma regarding the management of symptoms or conditions like cough, shortness of breath, and wheezing. By maintaining the health records and medical diagnosis, it becomes easy to cure asthma.

8.1. Summary of Key Points Discussed

First aid for an asthma attack involves a combination of techniques and the administration of the appropriate medications. If the person having the asthma attack has an inhaler, then he should be given between 1 and 6 puffs of his reliever inhaler (usually salbutamol or albuterol) every 15 to 20 minutes. If he does not have a prescribed inhaler and spacer, then he should be taken to the emergency as soon as possible for emergency medical care. If, on the other hand, the person's prescribed inhaler is not effective (he did not show improvement or he is getting worse, having an attack, or resting for the previous four hours and not taking his inhaler), he has to be instructed to take 10 to 20 puffs of his reliever inhaler and then to call for emergency medical care. While waiting for the ambulance, he can take up to 10 puffs every 4 hours. The casualty may use a single dose of a nebulizer. He or she will need mandatory medical attention if he or she does not begin to feel better very soon, or if he or she can take up to 10 puffs every hour of the bronchodilator.

This essay discusses first aid for an asthma attack, which can be provided in case the patient has an inhaler and in case he does not have an inhaler.

8.2. Emphasizing the Importance of Preparedness

According to coordination between GINA and NAEPP, we considered moderate asthma as moderate persistent asthma and vice versa. During any adversities like vomiting, heavy diarrhea or excessive abdominal cramps which may distract from your treatment, one should call the emergency department if experiencing heavy wheezing. Let your nose and mouth contribute during panic attacks. Breathe through your nose and exhale through the mouth. Panic takes away air from the abdomen. In a panic attack, say loudly, forceful and exhalation. The American College of Chest Physicians and the American Academy of Allergy and Immunology have recommended the activation of emergency medical services even in mild asthma.

Covid-19 has already highlighted the severity of the issue which comes with unpreparedness or dullness. The initiation of a fast service without any promise is not possible in the asthma condition. It is important to be ready and to take some precautionary measures which help you as a first aid as well as for long-term conditions. An asthma action plan (AAP) and regular follow-up help to give you a developed, hassle-free life. Asthma is characterized by bronchial hyperactivity or bronchial obstruction. It is a chronic inflammatory condition that could be severe, mild, moderate or persistent. It is characterized by quick-acting bronchospasm, constriction of vocal cords resulting in difficult breathing, coughing, chest tightening, and wheezing panic attack.

Preventing Asthma Attacks: A Comprehensive Guide

1. Introduction to Asthma Attacks

We hope that this guide will equip you with everything you need to know about preventing an asthma attack and that it will better prepare you to discuss this important medical topic with your doctor. If you have not yet received an asthma diagnosis but suspect that you may have the disease, we encourage you to consult with a medical professional to schedule appropriate testing. It is important to work closely with a doctor to prevent an asthma attack if you have already received an asthma diagnosis. This guide is based on evidence-based research and includes several illustrative case studies to further inform those diagnosed with asthma and those preparing for asthma-related medical consultation.

Welcome to our complete guide designed to provide you with everything you need to know in order to prevent asthma attacks. Throughout this guide, we will be covering a variety of topics related to the prevention of asthma attacks, from understanding the causes of an asthma attack to forming a comprehensive asthma attack prevention and maintenance plan with your doctor. In order to equip you with the most comprehensive knowledge base, we also cover the idea that it is sometimes not possible to prevent an asthma attack from occurring, despite our best intentions. Readers will find support from numerous case studies, real-world examples, and evidence-based practices within this guide to provide confidence and assurance that they are making the correct medical decisions and beginning the proper treatment plan. This is especially true for asthma patients who are aware of their diagnosis and want to be proactive in managing their symptoms and preventing a future attack.

1.1. Understanding Asthma

None of the individuals want to have to deal with their asthma symptoms, so it's best to prevent asthma attacks by learning how to minimize your risks and be proactive in managing your care. Part of the reason why Michael and David keep their inhalers with their kit at all times is because they may not realize until it's too late to treat their exacerbation that they were in the middle of an asthma attack, and breathing into it helps them know immediately if they need to reduce their activity or get help. To make sure you stay out of the hospital, or that you have enough medicine to treat your cold or flu, make sure you have an emergency care plan with your medical doctor and pay attention to how you are feeling.

Asthma symptoms can arise out of nowhere or at any age, as Emily can confirm, but they are more common in younger individuals. Because the airways are so inflamed, anything that causes the lungs to function harder makes it more challenging to breathe. Other asthma symptoms include coughing, wheezing, shortness of breath, or chest tightness. Generally, the symptoms that an asthma sufferer experiences are referred to as "exacerbations" or "asthma attacks." They can last for a few minutes or days.

Asthma is a respiratory condition in which airways become inflamed and constricted, obstructing air from reaching the lungs. It can range in terms of severity, frequency, and duration, and can be a minor annoyance or a severe problem. It is a lifelong condition. As of this time, Emily's mother has repeated it several times, but increasing numbers of people are able to manage their condition and decrease the likelihood of serious asthma attacks developing over time.

2. Risk Factors and Triggers

Allergens are environmental substances that cause asthma symptoms to develop. Infections, such as colds, sinus infections, and bronchitis, can also initiate the release of histamine and other inflammatory chemicals that restrict the airways. Medications, such as aspirin, Aleve, and a high dose of aspirin, can produce respiratory challenges. Moreover, intense emotional states such as crying or laughter release epinephrine, also referred to as a cloudburst, that heightens heart rate, relaxes airways, and shuts down inflammation in an overstimulated state. By familiarizing oneself with the various elements which contribute to an asthma attack, one can make informed decisions to reduce their likelihood. Preventative measures include flu vaccines, monitoring symptoms and upcoming weather, avoiding secondhand smoke and pollutants, staying free of food and environmental allergens, regularly cleaning spaces, washing hands, consulting a doctor on whether emergency medication is necessary, and exercising according to doctor recommendations.

Asthma attacks can occur unexpectedly. While the causes are personal, the possibility of having an asthma attack can be increased or decreased through understanding various risk factors and triggers. Risk factors do not cause asthma, but can determine whether symptoms become severe enough to require medication or hospitalization. Notable risk factors include insufficient primary care, living in low socioeconomic neighborhoods, and smoking. Like risk factors, certain irritants, allergens, infections, medications, and emotions can act as triggers for an asthma attack.

2.1. Common Triggers

Sports. Many sports produce something called histamines, which is known to cause bronchoconstriction.

Stress. People with asthma are more likely to have problems with their healthcare and may have PTSD. Extreme emotions can make breathing harder for people with asthma.

Pollutants in the air: perfume, cigarette or other smoke (even when it doesn't smell like smoke), air pollution.

Alcohol. While doctors and researchers don't exactly know why, some trigger asthma attacks in some patients. There may be something in the fermentation process that encourages the creation of chemicals that can cause asthma.

Cockroach + dust mites. These pests make the home into an informal site of employment for allergen producers. Measures for getting rid of them are included in a later section on home indoor asthma prevention strategies. The best solution to beat pet allergens, however, is cleaner indoor air per a recent study.

Foods. An allergic response to something eaten can exacerbate asthma symptoms.

Pets. These furry friends can be a major factor in severe asthma, reducing lung function and increasing the chance of airway obstruction. Dirty pets are worse, so bathing often can help. While dander is generally a problem, it can take up to two months for a change in pet management to translate into a reduction in asthma symptoms.

Typical asthma triggers can vary, but proper asthma care should include an especially fastidious, deliberate approach to controlling these. Here, we provide a list of the most common types of factors reported to cause asthma attacks. By considering these factors, asthma patients can identify what may be increasing their risk of both their respiratory distress symptoms and exacerbation.

3. Recognizing Early Warning Signs

Your peak flow gives you an idea of whether your air passages are open (green), getting a little narrowed (yellow), or quite swollen (red) long before you'd otherwise sense there was trouble on the way. There's a top number that you can hit a little above and a bottom number that you should not go below over several days of careful monitoring. It's particularly good for gauging the intensity of the inflammation. A cough probably reflects moderate swelling in your air tubes. It's also a good idea to inform everyone involved where your peak flow rates ought to be and when they need to take action. Try to record your best of three values, but don't stress yourself if you can't seem to blow out hard enough to get a big reading. All measurements taken at once are a reflection of whatever was going on for an instant. This isn't a competition.

Mild and severe asthma attacks can be headed off at the pass if you're watchful for early warning symptoms. People with asthma tend to know that something's wrong before the wheezing starts. They may feel out of sorts, irritable, or uncharacteristically quiet. You may get variable amounts of swelling in your lungs. This can mean things like a mild cough or merely the sensation of chest tightness. Some people notice only a vague headache at the very tip of their foreheads; others experience a classic little lump in their throat. A deeper cough without phlegm that lingers past a few days is a more certain early warning signal; it's sometimes misinterpreted as a sign of bronchitis or a cold. During consistent times or in specific situations, asthmatics sometimes sense that they haven't made their usual "best effort" in breathing. This is definitely an alert.

3.1. Symptoms and Indicators

Asthma is a disease of the lungs in which inflammation causes constriction of the airways, producing wheezing, coughing, difficulty breathing, chest tightness or pain, sleep disturbances, and endurance limitations. Asthmatics usually have "good days" and "bad days," directly affecting productivity and health-related quality of life. An asthma attack, also known as an episode, exacerbation, or flare-up, is the sudden or gradual worsening of one or more asthma symptoms and is of concern because it may lead to the virulence or severity of symptoms progressive to respiratory arrest (asphyxia) and possible death if not intervened and reversed. A strong asthmatic has one or more of the following symptoms of an impending attack beginning to appear within the past 24 hours or beginning soon: shortness of breath, feeling out of breath, chest tightness, coughing/sore throat, or wheezing.

Asthma management involves the use of medications and environmental controls to minimize symptoms. A successful asthma management program also includes avoiding those activities, exposures, or behaviors that trigger asthma symptoms to a manageable level or prevent them from occurring, and patient education to ensure that the appropriate techniques and medications are used. An important part of asthma management that is sometimes overlooked is asthmatic triad education. Members of the asthmatic triad include the patient, the patient's family, and supportive friends. The following guide provides an in-depth discussion of asthma and how to prevent an asthma attack before it starts.

4. Asthma Action Plans

The steps in the asthma action plan will be different for everyone. The healthcare provider who writes your asthma action plan will show you what you can do to avoid things that make your asthma worse, help you understand your asthma symptoms, and show you when your asthma is under good control. They will also help you get emergency care if you have an asthma attack. Your asthma action plan is just for you. It's based on your asthma severity, age, home, school, and work environment, and other important information. Your healthcare provider will help you complete your written plan and will give you a copy. Once your plan is done, you should read and understand it and fill out the patient part of your written plan. Then, your healthcare provider will make final decisions about what you should do and will fill out your part of the written plan. Now you're ready to start using your asthma action plan!

An asthma action plan is a coordinated plan developed with a healthcare provider that tells you what medicines you should take, when to take them, and what to do if you need emergency help. It shows your personal asthma information and describes your medicines. It also includes things like how to recognize when your asthma is getting worse so you can get help before you have an asthma attack. Asthma action plans can help you prevent asthma attacks, manage your asthma if you have an asthma attack, and reduce emergency room or urgent care visits because of asthma attacks. It's important for everyone who has asthma to have a written asthma action plan.

4.1. Components of an Action Plan

The national guidelines suggest that these components and/or details be included in a written plan. The action plan should be a guide to help diagnose disease or decide if another family member is the one having a problem, not a fixed script where the patient or family member cannot help to change a drug schedule or other care as the asthma changes. A copy of your asthma management plan and charts/instructions should be given to your healthcare provider if you or they do not already have a copy. This is particularly necessary for you to keep a copy of the notes on your medication, time for each medication, and also all prior written asthma treatment plans if you have had previous ones if you have an emergency visit to a new office.

Children may have additional information such as physical activity or school participation guidelines.

- Office visits to review the current medication needs - Specific symptoms that need an immediate call to a healthcare provider - Urgent care to seek for sudden changes in lung function, needing a rescue medicine more than every 4 hours at a time or the one appearing to be ineffective for your symptoms - A chart for peak flow monitoring, shot schedule, or allergy desensitization schedule.

An asthma management plan may also make suggestions or outline when to follow up with a doctor or update your plan, such as:

- Long-term control medicines for asthma (inhaled corticosteroids, long-acting beta2-agonists, leukotriene inhibitors, and others) - how much, how often, how to recognize most common side effects - Quick-relief asthma rescue medicine (also known as a fast-acting inhaler) that contains albuterol - how much and when to take it.

An effective asthma management plan typically will include components such as environmental control, trigger prevention, and, most importantly, a medication plan that outlines what schedule to follow for different types of asthma:

5. Medications and Treatment Options

4. Leukotriene Inhibitors: Work against leukotrienes, chemicals that are associated with the inflammation of the bronchial passages in individuals suffering from asthma. In 1998, the first leukotriene receptor antagonist was approved for use as a first-line treatment for asthma.

3. Xanthine Derivatives: Are used as bronchodilators and improve breathing. They are usually not the first choice for asthma treatment.

2. Corticosteroids: Taken daily, these medications either reduce inflammation and swelling or block the actions of the chemicals that cause inflammation and swelling. Without these changes, it is possible for asthma to recur. Inhaled corticosteroids are very common, though a number of other medications may be prescribed.

1. Bronchodilators: Divided into two types, these medications stop the spasms of the smooth muscles around the bronchial tubes and relieve symptoms. Some are long-acting and gradually increase the size of the bronchial passages, while others are short-acting and do the same quickly. Short-acting bronchodilators are used when a quick-relief bronchodilator is necessary.

Adapted from an original list by the National Heart, Lung, and Blood Institute (NHLBI), we have compiled a comprehensive review of the various types of medications and treatment options that exist for asthma prevention. It is likely that a combination of these pharmaceutical methods or therapeutic measures will be best for most people suffering from asthma. As a general rule, those medications geared toward preventing and controlling asthma are given every day. Those that are used to alleviate asthma symptoms should be used only when necessary. If your asthma is mild and/or infrequent, occasional doses should be all you require.

5.1. Types of Medications

3. Combination Medications If you are taking an inhaled steroid in combination with a reliever, it must be used for the purpose of both relieving symptoms and preventing symptoms. Taking a puff or two of a reliever and then taking a particular type of inhaled steroid can help to quickly open the airways significantly more than taking the reliever on its own if your asthma symptoms are not well controlled.

2. Relievers These medications are taken as needed to quickly open up the airways and relieve symptoms. They are also known as rescue medications. If your reliever is needed more than once a week (other than 5-15 minutes before exercise), it is usually a sign of poor asthma control.

1. Controllers These are medications to be taken on a daily basis to prevent asthma symptoms. They work by reducing the swelling in the airways and keeping them open, which in turn keeps the muscles from tightening. Careful use and regular monitoring of these medications are recommended for all asthmatics and are absolutely essential for those with persistently poor asthma control.

There are a number of types of medications used for the treatment of asthma. They work in different ways and may be taken in a number of ways. They may be taken by the mouth (orally) in the form of a syrup or a tablet, by inhalation, or by injection.

6. Lifestyle Modifications

Mold: It's imperative to clean mold as far as possible in your home. Use dehumidifiers and air conditioners to alleviate allergies. It's also recommended to wash your pet's water and food dishes weekly with warm water to kill mold.

Cockroach and insects: Cockroach and insect infestation can aggravate symptoms, so take every possible step to remove these crawling insects from your home.

Pets: If you are allergic to animal dander, you should avoid pets. If you previously had a pet and it led to an asthma attack, avoid being near that pet in the future.

Smoking: An asthma patient should not smoke or be in the environment of others' smoke. In fact, smoking is the most critical condition for treating asthma. In addition to causing asthma, smoking can make it increasingly difficult to keep asthma symptoms under control. You should also avoid both first and second-hand tobacco smoke. Use electric or gas ovens and stoves at home to lessen exposure to pollution caused by burning wood.

Exercise: Regular exercise is known to improve the quality of life in asthma patients. However, you should avoid extreme temperatures. On cold days, you can cover your nose and mouth with a scarf to help filter the air as you breathe it into your lungs.

Diet: Be mindful of your diet because it might determine your risk of suffering from asthma. For example, eating fast food three or more times a week may exacerbate the disease. Also, if you have obesity, it should be treated because it may enhance the risk of asthma.

In this way, exercise is a crucial factor in one's health. An individual's respiratory health can be increased over time with consistent, effective exercise. In fact, swimming is particularly beneficial as it is associated with controlled breathing. On the subject of controlled breathing, personal psychology can also be altered to remove anxiety triggers from an individual's life, thus reducing the risk of stressful, anxiety-induced asthma attacks. Nevertheless, without medications or other interventions from a licensed doctor, those with asthma always run a risk of an attack. Trainers should be cautious to note that overexertion can trigger an attack if they're not careful with their athletes. Similarly, varying degrees of inflammation should be taken into account, and athletes may need occasional reduced dosages of their medications to reduce the risk of an asthma attack.

Crucially, when dealing with asthma, one should acknowledge the impact of diet and exercise on their condition. These changes will not cure one of asthma, but they should significantly reduce the risk of having an attack. As such, it's recommended that those with asthma seek a diet high in vitamin D. Unfortunately, vitamin D is only found in a few different foods, like almonds and salmon, so supplementation may be necessary in some for adequate intake. Also, individuals with asthma may have more difficulty getting sufficient amounts of the vitamin D precursor from sun exposure alone, so outdoor exposure alone may not be sufficient. Still, sunlight remains the best source of vitamin D for many nutritionists. Balancing physical health, one should also always be cautious to balanced intake with exercise and diet, explained by research that has shown that excessive vitamin D through supplementation increases fractures, harms athletic ability, and increases the risk of a heart attack.

7. Environmental Control

Environmental changes on the global level include government-implemented air quality standards, advocacy campaigns (think secondhand smoke), and adherence to standards set by professional societies like the American Society of Heating, Refrigerating, and Air-Conditioning Engineers. Despite a lack of large, well-controlled research studies to endorse the use of certain environmental controls, there seems to be consensus among pulmonary physicians that implementing allergen- or trigger-reducing strategies in the home environment is a cornerstone of asthma management. The most frequently encountered issues for persons with asthma revolve around indoor air and containment of irritants. Some general recommendations include: Removing known agents such as animal dander, dust mites, and pollens that serve to trigger or exacerbate either allergic rhinitis and/or allergic asthma. Implementing irritant-reducing strategies, such as special vacuums and other equipment designed for finely divided particles, dehumidifiers, and proper ventilation that utilizes High Efficiency Particulate Air (HEPA) filters.

Your environment can have a big impact on asthma. Make your living space as allergy- and asthma-free as possible. How? A start in your home could include replacing carpeting with wood or linoleum, washing curtains rather than sending them to the dry cleaner, choosing blinds over drapes, and minimizing upholstery. But the clock doesn't stop at home. The local environment, work settings, and schools play a big role, too. Proper ventilation, air filtration, smoke-free zones, and policy changes help keep ambient living and working spaces asthma-friendly.

7.1. Creating an Asthma-Friendly Environment

There are many things a person can do at work and at home to bring about this change. In this section, the term home applies to any place a person lives and the term work refers to any place a person works. To prevent asthma attacks, it is important to find out what the triggers are for that person. It is equally important to keep all possible asthma triggers controlled and removed from the environment to the extent that it is possible to do so. Managing and controlling a person's environment may mean making changes to buildings, grounds, and equipment; creating new rules that everyone must follow; working together to create an asthma-friendly community; and training workers and residents about why and how to be asthma friendly.

At home or work, many people feel that they are able to relax and have a good time. However, for some people, certain environments can have the exact opposite effect. For those with asthma, a clean, comfortable environment can make a huge difference in preventing asthma attacks. The main goal of preventing asthma attacks is to make indoor and outdoor environments as asthma-friendly as possible. This section will help design environments to reduce the risk of asthma attacks and limit asthma symptoms. There are many things that contribute to creating an asthma-friendly environment. When planning an environment that reduces the risk of asthma attacks, it is important to develop a plan of action that will bring about the best results.

8. Emergency Response

When should more reliever medication be used even when things seem fine? • The amount of reliever inhaler medication or frequency should not regularly increase to above 10 "puffs" a day. When one is partially preventing an asthma attack, doing so numerously means that more reliever must be administered in order to reverse the narrowing of the airways. The serial peak flow readings should not be used. Time is of the essence. When experiencing severe asthma symptoms, rely on symptoms rather than peak flow data.

Action plan. Make sure that you or the person suffering has an asthma action plan that guides what to do when one has difficulty breathing. An action plan provides a guide that details which medications should be administered, when, and the required doses. Carry the supplies, which include a reliever inhaler, or create a folder with all the necessary paperwork in case of a visit to the emergency room. If assistance is required to retrieve the supplies and bring them to where you are, reach out to someone close. Call emergency services. If the signs are quickly deteriorating, if more reliever medication is necessary but not providing relief, or if shortness of breath and breathing difficulties prevent normal activities or speech routines, then emergency medical attention should be sought.

Allergen challenge: The allergen challenge can replicate several features of asthma, including attacks of wheezing and airflow obstruction and plasma leakage. Bronchial responsiveness: After bronchial challenge, the reduction in lung function can be measured as a separate diagnostic test. In addition to being the gold standard for the diagnosis of asthma, demonstration of increased bronchial responsiveness associates with accelerated decline in lung function, symptoms which lead to increased use of inhaled steroids, and higher healthcare costs. A variety of indirect tests have been developed to assess bronchial hyper-responsiveness. De Mettoraphan Use of the synthetic protease inhibitor N-(2-R,S-4-methoxyphenylsulfonyl)-3-phenylethyl- R. (2R,4S) 3-{chloro-4-[(3-fluoroybenzoxy) phenylsulfonyl]oxiranylmethyl}-4-phenylsulfonyl-2-oxo-tetrahydro-furan-carboxamide (SCH 160237) potently inhibits de Mottoraphoe activity ex vivo in human plasma. SCH 160237 is orally active in a human whole blood de Mettoraphoe model and may be of value when selecting an asthma drug in countries with scarce resources for asthma therapy, where severe asthma can be lethal and an additional weapon is urgently needed.

Severe attacks: Many people ignore the warning signs that they are having a severe or life-threatening asthma attack. During a severe attack, you may need to be hospitalized. For some people with a severe asthma attack, life-threatening asthma symptoms develop so quickly that no treatment can prevent them from dying. More and more is known now about asthma, and various countries have published evidence-based guidelines and treatment protocols. Here we detail the exact drug protocols for a severe asthma attack. Severe or life-threatening asthma attack is the most dangerous feature of not having asthma controlled. Knowing how to deal with severe attacks is vital - for you or for someone who is looking after you.

9. Preventive Measures

The following are tips for allergen avoidance that will help reduce exposure to common potential asthma triggers. Pets often have proteins in their saliva and scaly skin cells, known as dander, which can cause allergic reactions in some people. Cat allergens are generally airborne and can transfer from place to place, while dog allergens are generally not airborne. Some of these allergens found in pet saliva and dander can cause allergic reactions and aggravate asthma symptoms in some individuals. Some individuals may have more severe asthma and allergies or other related allergic conditions when they come in contact with animals. While some individuals are allergic to pet dander, other factors related to pets can also cause allergies. Clearing the air sufficiently of the pet allergens in your home can be difficult once a pet has lived there for years. Trying to find a new home for the cat could be recommended in severe cases, after which the home will be professionally cleaned of pet allergens. It is possible to keep a cat in the home even with significant pet allergies by being dedicated to avoidance measures.

Dust mites are a common trigger of asthma, especially for those with another condition called allergic rhinitis. Because asthma attacks can occur following exposure to allergens like dust mites or pollen, it is important to reduce dust mite exposure for those with an allergy.

9.1.3. Rodents • The allergen: Urine, dander, and saliva from mice and rats can prompt attacks. • Plugging up holes and decreasing potential food supplies can help avoid infestations. Outside traps may help keep rodent numbers down.

9.1.2. Cockroaches • The allergen: Waste, saliva, body parts, and eggs are the culprits when it comes to cockroach allergens. • Pesticides and traps can eliminate cockroaches, and bait gel may be convenient. Fixing leaks and holes is important because cockroaches need water and hiding spots to live.

9.1.1. House Dust Mites • The allergen: Proteins produced by house dust mites and found in their feces. There are at least 23 proteins known to trigger allergic reactions in humans. • Allergy-proof bedding and pillowcases can keep symptoms at bay while sleeping. If that's not an option, there are a variety of in-home methods to kill the mites or get rid of their feces. • Dust-trapping mats and throw rugs should be removed to limit the presence of the mites.

Identifying allergens that can trigger attacks and finding ways to reduce exposure are central to preventing asthma. While there is no definitive guide for allergen avoidance, we salute the researchers, clinicians, and patients who have collected this wealth of experience. For each major asthma trigger, we present what the relevant allergen is and how to avoid it.

10. Managing Asthma in Different Age Groups

We cannot just look at them differently; we have to experience everything in the different ages of the children and young people with asthma. With babies, asthma management with inhalers is trickier. Toddlers and older parents need to monitor when their children secretly have a low dose of steroid inhaler. This intermediate level text presents detailed guidance on how to manage children with asthma in primary care from 2019. Adolescent asthma care and management are unique; asthma is least well pronounced when children are small, and children adapt to it gradually. Parents may have little experience of symptoms of asthma in their children when at a young age. You're the healthcare professional who has designed a framework for managing asthma in children and a common approach to providing education and treatment, as described in the 2019 BTS/SIGN Adult Guideline.

Managing asthma often becomes problematic as children grow, and the challenges do not diminish with puberty. Then, in adulthood, some may exhibit symptoms for the first time. The involvement of families, school staff, and healthcare professionals of various types becomes increasingly necessary as adolescence begins. Involve people, practices, and services that are go-to figures for them, such as college healthcare services, different residential services, or employment providers. It is essential to manage asthma by acknowledging the transitions of the patients and their families and the difficulties faced by the healthcare professionals associated with them. In the same way, schools are asked to support establishment absences for children with asthma. So, at university, adjustments may be required for illness during periods of exams and coursework.

10.1. Children with Asthma

The treatment of childhood asthma is similar to that of adults. The youngest children often require "extra help" in getting their medication to their lungs. This can be done by utilizing a spacer/holding chamber or a nebulizer. The proper medication, at the correct dose, is essential in controlling both daily asthma and flare-ups. There are also rescue medications that work by relaxing the bands around the air passages, like the bands in blood pressure cuffs, so that the airways can open up and are not squeezed too tight. Preventive or anti-inflammatory medications help calm and return the lining of the inflamed airways to normal. The most commonly used anti-inflammatory medications are steroids which are not the same as the performance-enhancing drugs abused by athletes. Steroids used for treating asthma have minimal side effects, especially when inhaled at appropriate doses described by the physician.

Children with asthma have certain needs and face special considerations that adults do not. The most important thing a parent can do is to develop a good management plan for their child and communicate closely with healthcare providers. By continuously monitoring and adjusting the management plan, parents can nip problems in the bud. Children's asthma is constantly changing; therefore, their management plan will change as well. It is best to be seen more often by the healthcare provider in the beginning so that they may better control or manage the child's asthma. Parents need to watch for the "HUFFS and PUFFS" of asthma that might indicate they would need to seek emergency care. Also, taking preventive measures with the child's environment, i.e. home, school, can prevent flare-ups resulting in asthma attacks and lung damage.

11. Future Developments and Research

Our understanding of airway inflammation in asthma is rapidly evolving. Now, various cytokines and chemokines are recognized as drivers and amplifiers of inflammatory reactions, and as such, represent potential targets for future therapeutic intervention. Moreover, the complexity of asthma pathogenesis means that the potentially important targets are not limited only to those that could lead to the inhibition of mediator release from activated cells. The possibility of identifying pharmacologic substances that exert an antagonistic effect on more than one factor associated with the initiation or amplification of the disease process is also evident.

Methylxanthines such as theophylline/aminophylline can provide the benefit of maximum bronchodilation over long periods, but are not regarded as necessary when the prevention of bronchial hyperreactivity is our goal. Inhaled corticosteroids are useful for controlling lung inflammation, but their use can be associated with systemic side effects. Treatment with ketotifen is a safe and cost-effective approach, due to its capacity of preventing the onset of inflammation via a dual mechanism of action. Research on the above-mentioned topic has given birth to the discovery of leukotriene receptor inhibitors. A promising advancement on the research and development front for the inhibition of internal mediator release is the description of phosphodiesterase type 4 by a team of investigators. The importance of cholinergic innervation in asthma is clear, and thus, the potential use of the class of cholinesterase inactivators that achieve their inhibitory action selectively on acetylcholinesterase in its therapeutic potential should be acknowledged.

11.1. Innovations in Asthma Management

One advance that can help in the prevention of severe upper respiratory illnesses is the prevention or treatment of viral diseases. In the pipeline, there are monoclonal antibody treatments that, once we become infected with a cold virus, can decrease the length of time and severity of symptoms by approximately 50%. The trial to investigate the preventative use of this treatment in people who have mucus-hypersecretion is underway, and we should know the results in approximately 2 years. There are also people researching how the bacteria that normally live in our nose interact with cold viruses and why some people get really sick when they get a cold. They have found that people with asthma might not have good bacteria in their nose and may have bad bacteria present, leading to more severe asthma symptoms and a longer recovery from viral infections. These researchers are exploring whether giving people good bacteria could protect them from developing viral-induced asthma attacks.

Lifestyle and environmental management are critical in controlling symptoms and preventing attacks. Ensuring good air quality indoors is important, as is addressing other allergic or irritant triggers. The use of immunotherapies in various forms to help overcome environmental allergies is also being offered by specialists. Interesting innovations in the world of asthma management are coming up. The potential of some of these new approaches and technologies is very exciting and could be a real part of the solutions for prevention and treatment in the future.

12. Conclusion and Key Takeaways

This guide provides you with tools to prepare for and take control of your asthma triggers. These proactive steps range from basic housekeeping to advanced indoor environmental quality (IEQ) services that can help you make smart decisions and measures to protect your home and, most importantly, your loved ones. The guide has covered the tips and tricks of asthma management, and we hope you've learned something new about how to protect yourself and your family from the unexpected trauma of an asthma attack. Key takeaways: - Triggers are classified as indoor or outdoor, both of which can lead to an asthma attack. - Immunotherapy (allergy shots) can train your immune system to tolerate allergens that may otherwise trigger your asthma. - Smoke, while not as deadly as allergens, is a common irritant that contributes to asthma symptoms. - A peak flow meter can measure the inflammation in your lungs, acting as the same test that caused your doctor to diagnose you with asthma in the first place.

Managing asthma to prevent attacks is a proactive process. With the appropriate tools and information, you can control your condition and avoid asthma attacks. Good asthma management starts with a thorough understanding of your individual triggers and the allergens and irritants that put you at risk. Over time, develop a strong relationship with the medical professionals who treat you. Communicate your symptoms and their severity, and always share your personal experiences with any medications you are taking. If you sense that a particular treatment or inhaler is not providing you with much relief, discuss it with your healthcare provider and consider adjustments or alternatives.